Between Hope and Action

ISBN (Digital Version): 979-8-89758-000-2

ISBN (Print-on-Demand): 979-8-89758-001-9

Published by Spanish Language 4 Business.

Dedication

To my wife, my tireless companion, whose support never wavered, even when my decisions seemed to defy the reality of the moment—only for time to prove them right. Thank you for your infinite patience, your unwavering faith, and for walking with me every step of this adventure called life.

To my son, with the hope that each story inspires him to reflect, learn, and face challenges with determination. May he always value the power of ideas and the importance of forging his own path with wisdom and strength.

To my dear father, a guide and source of strength in the key moments of my life. His advice and support have been my greatest foundation.

To my mother, who embarked on the journey to eternal life when I was a child. Though I have few memories of her, I have always felt her protection in every moment of my life.

Prologue

I have always admired those who dedicate themselves to writing, not only for their mastery of language and expertise but for their ability to convey ideas with creativity and clarity. I never imagined that I would one day write a book myself, but technological advancements have made once-unattainable projects more accessible.

At its core, this book explores how political and influential leaders' decisions shape society. Addressing corruption, greed, and unchecked ambition is essential for building a fairer, more prosperous system, particularly in areas as vital as healthcare.

This is a work of fiction and does not depict real people or events. The characters and situations are entirely imaginary, and any resemblance to actual individuals or occurrences is purely coincidental.

The story also carries a personal touch. The choice of the city of San Quirino was inspired by my middle name, which I inherited from my great-great-grandfather. During a recent trip to Italy—a country I deeply admire for its rich culture and warm people—I discovered its Italian roots, and a town called San Quirino. This connection led me to set part of the story there as a symbolic tribute.

José Quirino

Table of Contents

Part One:

The Awakening of a Cause

The Dawn of a Purpose

"Progress is impossible without change, and those who cannot change their minds cannot change anything."
— George Bernard Shaw

The sunrise bathed the fief of San Quirino in golden hues, illuminating the hills and the majestic Castle of the Lily, the ancestral home of the Marquises of Varenti. From the terrace, the young Baron Aldemar de Varenti gazed at the slowly awakening landscape. The village cottages, humble and scattered, were still shrouded in the soft morning mist, while the first sounds of the day began to fill the air: the clanging of the blacksmith's hammer, the bleating of sheep, and the voices of peasants heading to the fields.

The castle, with its towers and thick walls, was a symbol of the power of the Varenti family, led by Marquis Severino de Varenti and Marchioness Isabella de Varenti. For generations, they had ruled this region of northern Italy with a firm hand. In a world where the Renaissance blossomed with art, science, and thought in cities like Florence and Venice, San Quirino remained trapped in immutable feudal structures. The peasants worked the land with resignation, paying tributes that sustained the nobles' luxury, while the latter watched from their high walls, clinging to traditions that seemed eternal.

Aldemar, however, did not share such a vision. Unlike his older brother, Count Aldric de Varenti, a celebrated warrior whose exploits were immortalized in songs and frescoes in the family chapel, Aldemar did not seek military glory. Educated in the castle by monks, he had developed a natural affinity for the healing sciences. Spending entire days studying treatises on botany and medicine, he would dissect plants in search of remedies for the villagers' ailments.

However, it was not only in books that Aldemar found solace. From a young age, he had cultivated an exceptional skill with the bow and arrow, a talent that few in the castle fully knew. For Aldemar, archery was not merely an exercise in strength but an art in which the mind and body worked in perfect harmony.

As the cool morning breeze tousled his dark brown hair, his hazel eyes, watchful yet weary, rested on the village. There, a group of peasants moved slowly, tools slung over their shoulders, resigned to the daily grind. Aldemar watched them with a mix of compassion and frustration. His visits to the village had revealed the hidden reality: men and women weakened by fever, emaciated children, and elders barely enduring yet another winter. Diseases, fueled by poor living conditions, were treated just enough to keep them working. Never healed. Never freed.

Meanwhile, the Council of Physicians, an alliance of wealthy healers backed by the Most Serene Republic of Venice and led by the arrogant Duke Lorenzo Malvini, along with his good friend Marquis Travius of the Hills, held a monopoly on medicine in the region. Their remedies, exorbitantly priced, served only to mask symptoms and perpetuate the cycle of illness and exploitation. Aldemar felt that his family, with its opulence and indifference, was part of the problem.

In his room, a worn wooden table was covered with scribbled papers and a botanical treatise brought by a merchant from Venice. He had spent the night studying ways to relieve a fever affecting several children in the village, including Marielle, whose health was worsening by the moment. Aldemar knew his efforts would not change the fate of all afflicted, but saving one life was an act significant enough.

The sound of boots echoed behind him, pulling him out of his thoughts. Aldric appeared on the terrace, his gleaming armor reflecting the first rays of sunlight.

"Daydreaming again, brother?" Aldric asked with a lopsided smile, a mix of teasing and affection.

Aldemar raised his hands, showing the green herbal stains on his fingers.

"Guilty," he replied calmly. "I was preparing a salve for Marielle; her fever hasn't improved."

Aldric looked at him with disguised admiration.

"You worry too much, Aldemar. These people are stronger than you think. You can't save everyone."

Aldemar fixed his gaze on the horizon.

"I can't save everyone, but I can save someone. And sometimes, that's enough."

Before Aldric could respond, the commanding voice of their father, Marquis Severino de Varenti, thundered from inside:

"Aldemar! To my study, now!"

Aldric exchanged a warning look with his brother. Aldemar removed his leather apron and, smoothing out his tunic, stained with oil and dirt, headed toward the study. The worn boots he wore betrayed his long walks to the village—a detail that deeply irritated Severino.

The study was a sanctuary of power: heavy curtains, shelves filled with account books, and an imposing desk that dominated the room. Severino, with his rigid posture and stern gaze, wasted no time speaking.

"You are a noble, Aldemar, the second son of this house. Yet you insist on squandering your time with peasants and herbs."

Aldemar held his father's gaze.

"Is it not the duty of a ruler to care for his people? After all, a castle without a foundation cannot stand."

Severino's eyes narrowed.

"They work because they must. That is their place. Ours is to rule."

Aldemar took a deep breath.

"Healthy and prosperous people strengthen the fief, Father. Knowledge and justice are not signs of weakness but of progress."

The silence weighed heavily in the room. Finally, Severino commanded,

"Tomorrow, you will attend the Council. It is time for you to learn the duties expected of you."

Aldemar nodded stiffly and left, but deep down, he knew his path did not lie in the cold halls of the Marquess's Council. His destiny was in the fields of San Quirino, alongside his people.

The sun had fully risen, illuminating every corner of the fief. As he gazed at the village from the terrace, Aldemar silently vowed that he would not rest until he had built a future where justice and knowledge formed the foundation of his home. Perhaps, one day, his compassion, determination, and skill with the bow would become weapons in the fight for the dignity of those without a voice.

Change, he thought, began with a single just act.

The Spark of Change

One day, as Baron Aldemar de Varenti returned from one of his visits to the village, he was intercepted by an older man on the dirt road. The figure, dressed in a dark tunic and holding a finely carved wooden staff, was unmistakable: Baron Nicandro, the medical advisor, one of the most respected members of the Council of Physicians.

Known for his severe appearance and silent interventions at Council meetings, many regarded him as untouchable, firmly aligned with the rules of the Most Serene Republic of Venice and the practices of conventional medicine.

"Baron Aldemar," Nicandro greeted firmly, leaning on his intricately carved staff as he fixed his gaze on him. "I have been hearing about your... activities for quite some time now."

Aldemar stopped, frowning as the breeze swirled dry leaves around them.

"My activities are merely an attempt to alleviate the suffering of those without resources," Aldemar replied, his tone calm yet resolute.

Nicandro let out a faint, sarcastic laugh and shook his head.

"Boy, you don't know what you're doing," the old man said, his tired gray eyes locked firmly on Aldemar. "I know how it feels. When I was young, I had the same ideas. I saw injustice, suffering, and thought I could change it. But the world doesn't work that way."

For a fleeting moment, Aldemar noticed a spark of nostalgia in Nicandro's eyes.

"Well, why didn't you try?" Aldemar asked, stepping closer to him.

Nicandro gripped his staff tightly.

"Because uncertainty weighs heavier than comfort. Challenging traditions means losing everything: stability, respect, the safety of a quiet life. I thought I could survive on principles, but I was wrong," he admitted quietly, as though confessing a sin.

Aldemar looked at him with a mix of astonishment and growing sadness.

"And now? Do you live peacefully knowing that suffering persists?"

Nicandro narrowed his eyes, and after a moment of silence, his voice regained its usual firmness.

"I'm not here to talk about my past. I'm here to warn you, Baron Aldemar," he said, pointing a finger at him. "What you are doing with your free remedies and prevention talks is disrupting the Council. The peasants speak of you, trusting your remedies more than ours. Do you understand how dangerous that is?"

Aldemar crossed his arms, a defiant gesture toward the elder.

"If my actions are dangerous, it is because they expose the greed of a broken and corrupted system. It's not the remedy that threatens your business, Nicandro, but the truth."

The old physician drew a deep breath, as though trying to keep his composure.

"You have a noble heart, but your vision is naive. This truth you speak of will not lead you to justice but to ruin. The Council does not forgive those who challenge its authority. It wouldn't be the first time an idealist loses his head." Nicandro paused, letting his words sink in. "Think carefully about what you're doing, young man. There's no turning back on this path."

Aldemar held the old man's gaze, unflinching.

"You're afraid because the weight of your decisions has crushed you, Nicandro. But I cannot stand idly by."

Nicandro studied him for a long moment, his expression unreadable, though something in his gaze hinted at a sliver of respect, perhaps even envy. Finally, he turned and began to walk away, his hunched figure gradually disappearing down the path.

"Don't say I didn't warn you," the old man muttered before vanishing among the trees.

Aldemar remained silent, the wind stirring his tunic as he pondered Nicandro's words. He knew the old man was not lying: defying the Council was a tremendous risk, albeit a necessary act. The suffering of his people had ignited a fire within him that could not be extinguished.

With renewed determination, Aldemar returned to the village that afternoon, resolute in continuing his work. Nicandro embodied the very thing he feared becoming: someone who, out of fear, had abandoned their fight. And Aldemar would not allow fear to dictate his path.

The Price of Truth

"Truth is the only solid ground upon which men can walk without falling."
— William Faulkner

The Council of Physicians wasted no time reacting. The growing support that Baron Aldemar de Varenti was receiving among the peasants posed a direct threat to their authority and, more importantly, their profits. For weeks, rumors of his generosity and knowledge of preventive medicine had traveled from the fields to neighboring villages, spreading unease among the Council members.

Gathered in the Hall of Twelve Lamps, a dark and opulent chamber in the residence of Grand Duke Vittorio of Astelari, the Council members deliberated tensely. Duke Lorenzo Malvini, the leader of the Council of Physicians, slammed his fist on the table, his voice resonating with authority.

"This insolent boy is undermining our prestige and, worse, our profits," he said coldly, his gaze sweeping across those present. "Free remedies, advice on hygiene... Since when do peasants have the right to such luxuries? What this young man is doing is not only foolish but a betrayal of his class."

Murmurs of approval rippled through the room. Only Baron Nicandro, seated in the back with his face shadowed, remained silent. He listened to every word, though the lines of worry on his brow betrayed an internal conflict.

"He must be stopped," Duke Malvini continued. "If he does not silence himself voluntarily, we will force him to. He will be offered two options: silence... or exile."

Nicandro finally raised his gaze.

"Are you certain about this?" His voice, though soft, carried a weight that made the others turn to him. "Aldemar is no nameless peasant. He's a noble—a Varenti."

The duke shot him a withering glare.

"That is precisely why his betrayal is doubly unforgivable. If a noble challenges our practices, what will stop the peasants from following his example? Discipline must be maintained."

Nicandro pressed his lips together and nodded, aware that any further words might be interpreted as sympathy toward Aldemar.

A messenger was summoned that very night and sent to the Castle of the Lily, the residence of Marquis Severino de Varenti, carrying a scroll sealed with the emblem of the Council.

At dawn, Baron Aldemar de Varenti was in the castle's library when a servant handed him the letter. Breaking the seal, he read the words with a furrowed brow and clenched lips:

Baron Aldemar de Varenti: Cease immediately your activities that disrupt the order of the fief. Should you persist, you will be exiled from San Quirino for treason against your class.

Indignation coursed through him. At that moment, the library doors burst open, and his father stormed in, his face flushed with fury.

"I warned you, Aldemar! Your stubbornness has brought disgrace upon our house! Do you understand what you've done?" Severino roared, snatching the letter from Aldemar's hands and, in a rage, hurling it to the floor as though it burned him.

Aldemar rose to his feet, his hazel eyes shining with a resolve that matched his father's tempest.

"All I have done is fulfill my duty to those who depend on us. Is it not a noble's responsibility to ensure the well-being of their people?"

"Enough!" Severino thundered, his voice booming like a storm. "You will remain silent and put an end to this madness—or you will renounce your name and your home!"

Silence engulfed the room for a moment. Aldemar took a deep breath before responding,

"I would rather lose my title and my home than my conscience, Father. The truth cannot be silenced."

After staring at his son with disbelief and disdain, Marquis Severino de Varenti turned on his heel and left the room without uttering another word. Aldemar was left alone, and within him, an irrevocable decision had been made. He knew that defying the Council of Physicians would not only jeopardize his position but also his life.

From that day, the shadow of exile began to loom over him, but he also felt a renewed strength. Baron Aldemar de Varenti swore to himself that if the price of truth was to lose everything, he would pay it willingly.

Between Duty and Doubt

"The real voyage of discovery consists not in seeking new landscapes,
but in having new eyes."
— Marcel Proust

Silence enveloped the gardens of the Castle of the Lily. Beneath the shelter of the cypresses, Baron Aldemar de Varenti pulled his bowstring with automatic movements. The string vibrated with a clear, almost musical sound as arrows flew through the air, striking the target with unerring precision. Yet his mind was elsewhere.

"Again!" he muttered to himself, drawing the bowstring tighter.

Practice after practice, Aldemar sought to quell the storm of thoughts that haunted him. He reflected on Baron Nicandro's words—his warnings and confessions. Were Nicandro's steps in his youth so different from his own? Uncertainty, the fear of failure and losing everything, weighed on him like a stone. He knew what he faced was immense: a reality built over centuries, a way of life accepted and defended by those who benefited from it.

At night, he continued experimenting with plants. The process of crafting new salves and medicinal mixtures served as both a distraction and a reminder that his work could not stop. Yet each breakthrough brought up the same question: was it worth risking everything for something that could be crushed by an unyielding system?

One afternoon, his mother, Marchioness Isabella de Varenti, found him in the gardens. She was an elegant woman, her dark hair framing a face marked by the serenity only years could bring. Her movements, delicate and measured, contrasted with the tension she saw in her son.

"Aldemar." Her voice was soft but firm, like a gentle caress laden with reproach. "Son, you must stop."

Aldemar lowered his bow and looked at her seriously. The wind lightly moved his mother's dress as she walked toward him, her face serene yet filled with worry.

"Mother, if you knew what I see out there, you'd understand why I can't," he argued, his tone a mix of fatigue and determination.

Isabella sighed before standing beside her son, gazing at the horizon beyond the castle walls.

"I understand more than you think, my son. When I was young, I too believed the world could be changed by sheer will. But what you're doing endangers not only your life but also the balance that sustains our position, our safety... our family."

Aldemar turned to her, his brow furrowed.

"Balance, Mother? It's a balance that only benefits a few while condemning so many. I cannot remain within these walls, pretending I don't see it."

Isabella looked at him with sadness, as if she saw a reflection of herself. Taking her son's hands into her own, she noticed the herbal stains and the roughness of work unbefitting a noble.

"Find another way, Aldemar," she said gently, her voice trembling slightly. "There are ways to help without directly challenging what surrounds us. The way our world works cannot be broken in an instant—not with impulses, not with a solitary fight."

Aldemar averted his gaze, letting his mother's words sink in. Was this what Nicandro had felt? The same internal struggle between the desire to act and the weight of consequences? Was it fear of failure that had silenced the old physician?

He reflected on Nicandro's warnings, on how the world can crush the dreams of idealists, leaving them as shadows of what they once aspired to be.

"I can't," he finally whispered, his voice barely audible. "I can't ignore it, Mother."

Pressing her lips together, Isabella gently released his hands and nodded. While hoping for a different answer, she knew Aldemar was as steadfast as his father in his decisions, though their paths differed.

"Just think carefully," she implored, walking away with the same elegance with which she had arrived. "If this is your battle, be sure you're ready for the price."

Aldemar watched her leave and, once alone, raised his bow again. He drew the string and fired, over and over, as if each arrow could unravel the tangled web of thoughts tormenting him.

Between tension, silence, and sleepless nights, he continued his work with plants, seeking new combinations of remedies as if the act of mixing herbs could also yield answers to his dilemmas.

He knew his mother was right about the consequences, yet he also knew that stopping was not an option.

Part Two:

The Struggle in the Shadows

A Pact in the Shadows

"Men are not united by their similarities, but by their common goals."
— Henry Ford

After weeks of uncertainty, Baron Aldemar de Varenti made his decision. He resumed his visits to the village, although with extreme caution. He preferred the dim light of dawn or the cover of night to reach the humble cottages of the peasants. Once there, he would treat ailments with simple remedies while sharing his knowledge of medicinal herbs and basic care. He knew that what he was doing was not only dangerous but deeply subversive.

"This is for you, but also for those who may need it in the future," he would say as he applied ointments or explained how to prepare a tea to reduce fever. "If anyone else finds out, it could mean the end of all this."

The peasants, grateful, listened attentively and promised to stay quiet. Aldemar saw hope and relief in their eyes, which only strengthened his determination. Still, he knew that even the smallest rumor of his continued work could spread like wildfire. Despite his best efforts to maintain secrecy, word of mouth—however discreet—eventually reached the wrong ears.

Baron Nicandro, the medical advisor, was one of the first to hear. The news of Aldemar's activities reached him just as he had convinced himself that the young noble had finally abandoned his crusade. A mix of frustration and curiosity compelled him to seek him out.

One night, after ensuring he wasn't being followed, Nicandro set out for the most remote part of the village. He found Aldemar in one of the farthest cottages, bent over an elderly woman as he ground herbs in a mortar. Through a small window, Nicandro watched as Aldemar gave the woman clear and careful instructions on how to administer the remedy. He waited for the young man to leave before intercepting him on the path.

The full moon illuminated Nicandro's face as he stood before Aldemar with a stern expression.

"You can't stop yourself, can you?" Nicandro said, his tone wavering between resignation and admiration.

Aldemar, surprised by the encounter, paused but remained calm. Knowing this moment was inevitable, he met the old man's gaze with determination etched on his face.

"I can't," he replied firmly. "If I close my eyes, it feels like I'm betraying something greater than myself."

Nicandro studied him intently, as if searching for something in his words. Finally, he sighed, running a hand through his graying hair.

"You're stubborn, boy. But also brave. Do you understand how dangerous this is?" he asked, though his tone of reproach was softer than it had been.

"I do. But you also know it's the right thing to do," Aldemar replied with a faint smile, trying to ease the tension.

The old man remained silent for a long moment, his expression a mixture of exhaustion and contemplation. Finally, he let out a heavy sigh, one that seemed to carry years of decisions and regrets.

"Fine," he conceded with a tone of resignation. "But if I'm going to help you, we do this on my terms. No one must know I'm involved. My position in the Council... cannot be jeopardized."

Aldemar nodded, knowing that even this small gesture of support was a victory.

"Thank you, Nicandro. This means more than I can express."

Nicandro shook his head, though a glimmer of respect flickered in his eyes. Under the light of the moon, the two men shook hands, sealing a clandestine pact that would bind their fates.

From that night on, Nicandro began sharing with Aldemar knowledge and resources that were otherwise beyond his reach. He provided access to more complex ingredients, advice on serious illnesses, and, most importantly, a network of contacts who could help without arousing suspicion.

While Aldemar worked in the shadows, Nicandro wrestled with his own conscience. Each time he helped the young noble, he felt as though he was defying the foundations of the system that had sustained him all his life. Yet, deep down, he knew there was something inherently just in what they were doing.

Bound by a common goal but from different paths, Aldemar and Nicandro began to challenge a system that seemed immovable. Their actions—small but significant—became a beacon of hope for those without a voice. Though danger constantly loomed over them, both knew that change would eventually demand a greater sacrifice.

For now, the struggle continued in the shadows.

The Catalyst of Rebellion

"Courage doesn't always roar; sometimes it's the quiet voice
at the end of the day saying: I will try again tomorrow."
— Mary Anne Radmacher

It was a cold, gray morning, with dawn barely illuminating the hills surrounding San Quirino. Baron Aldemar de Varenti, wrapped in his cloak, had set out early to visit one of the most distant villages in the fief. His ever-watchful gaze sought signs of the illnesses that had recently plagued the peasants, while his mind dwelled on the steps he needed to take to face the mounting danger.

The dirt paths were damp with dew, and the air smelled of fresh grass. As he crossed a low hill, he spotted a hunched figure by a well in the distance. At first glance, it seemed to be just another peasant, but the man's movements were hurried and furtive. As Aldemar approached, he noticed that the man, dressed in dark clothes and wearing a hat that partially concealed his face, was pouring a thick substance into the water.

Suddenly, an elderly woman appeared with a basket in her hands and shouted in a trembling voice: "Hey! What are you doing?"

The man flinched and, upon seeing Aldemar approaching, dropped the container and fled into the forest. "Stop! Halt!" Aldemar shouted as he unstrung his bow and nocked an arrow.

The fugitive ran swiftly, but Aldemar, with his characteristic precision, fired. The arrow flew cleanly and struck the man's thigh, sending him tumbling to the ground with a cry of pain.

Rushing over and grabbing the man by the collar, Aldemar shoved him against a tree and demanded answers.

"Speak! What were you doing at the well?"

"I—I don't know what you're talking about!" the man gasped, trembling with fear and pain.

Aldemar shoved him again, his gaze burning with fury.

"I saw what you did! Tell me who sent you and why you poisoned the water!"

The man, his eyes wide with terror, finally confessed:

"I—it was Marquis Travius of the Hills… he and Duke Lorenzo Malvini … they paid me to do it. Poisoning the water makes people sick, and they sell the remedies. They make money… lots of money."

The echo of those words reverberated in Aldemar's mind. Poisoning the water to profit from suffering! He took a deep breath to contain his rage. With precise movements, he broke the arrow lodged in the man's thigh and improvised a tourniquet from a piece of his cloak.

"This is so you don't bleed out. It's not for you—my fight isn't with you," he said coldly, then handed the man a makeshift staff for support. "Now go. If you try something like this again, you won't be so lucky."

The man, nodding frantically, limped away before disappearing into the trees. Aldemar returned to the poisoned well, staring at it in silence. He knew this was just the beginning of something much larger. His fists clenched tightly. He could not allow such a thing to happen again. From that moment on, he vowed to watch over the nearby wells and began considering how to organize the peasants to protect them from future poisonings.

The sun began to peek over the hills. As Aldemar made his way back to the castle, his mind was already weaving plans. Baron Nicandro, the medical advisor, needed to be informed, and this time Aldemar wouldn't just seek evidence but also allies to expose the Council's corruption.

Marquis Travius of the Hills and Duke Lorenzo Malvini had taken their greed too far, and Aldemar knew the next confrontation would be even more dangerous.

That night, after returning to the castle following hours of treating and advising the villagers, Aldemar's resolve was unshaken. However, he understood that his actions would not only endanger himself but also his family. If he continued living under the roof of the Marquises of Varenti, the Council's reprisals could endanger both his mother and brother.

The Silent Escape

With the weight of his decision heavy on his shoulders, Baron Aldemar de Varenti discreetly packed his belongings. Under the cover of darkness, he left the Castle of the Lily. No one saw him go. He walked for hours until he reached the humble cottage of a peasant on the outskirts of the fief. There, he found refuge, grateful for the hospitality of the man who recognized and accepted him without asking questions.

From this hideout, Aldemar began to plan his next move. He would immediately seek out Baron Nicandro to inform him of the recent events. The old physician, with his connections within the Council, could be a crucial ally in exposing the corruption of Marquis Travius of the Hills and Duke Lorenzo Malvini. However, before reaching out to him, Aldemar needed to ensure that the well and other village resources were protected.

The cottage became his new operations center. From there, he organized the peasants to guard the wells and explained the situation so they could remain vigilant. Delving deeper each day into his challenge, he was fully aware that his decision to leave home was irreversible.

Gazing at the horizon, Aldemar knew he had sacrificed the safety of his former life for a greater purpose. Now, with humble allies and a growing plan in his mind, the fight continued.

The Sacrifice in the Square

"The future belongs to those who believe in the beauty of their dreams."
— Eleanor Roosevelt

The months following the discovery of the crimes of Marquis Travius of the Hills and Duke Lorenzo Malvini brought palpable change to the affected villages.

Working in secrecy, Baron Aldemar de Varenti and Baron Nicandro had successfully prevented further contamination of the wells and improved the villagers' health. With lessons on hygiene, natural remedies, and constant vigilance of water sources, both children and adults began to recover. Misery slowly gave way to hope.

Nicandro, meanwhile, worked tirelessly. He had gathered irrefutable evidence of the Council's corruption. Among the evidence were sales records of the medicines, showing how they had been specifically directed to villages affected by the contamination; empty bottles with traces of the chemicals poured into the wells; and, most damning, secret correspondence between Travius and Malvini discussing plans to expand their scheme to neighboring fiefs. These letters, obtained through one of Nicandro's contacts within the Council, sealed the guilt of the villains.

Resistance grew stronger by the day. Inspired by the actions of Aldemar and Nicandro, the villagers began organizing more actively, aware that change also depended on them.

Meanwhile, the corruption at the highest levels was on the verge of being exposed, and the tension in San Quirino was as thick as the air before a storm.

The Confrontation in the Square

"Heroes don't always carry swords; sometimes they only carry the truth."
— Anonymous

The long-awaited Feast of Our Lady of the Rosary had finally arrived. The streets of San Quirino were alive with color and energy, as villagers and nobles gathered to celebrate. Garlands hung from windows, church bells rang out, and the air was filled with the aroma of freshly baked bread and simmering stews. Yet beneath the festive surface, an invisible tension loomed over the town.

Baron Aldemar de Varenti and Baron Nicandro had been planning this pivotal moment for weeks. After long discussions and careful preparation, they agreed that Nicandro would publicly confront Marquis Travius of the Hills and Duke Lorenzo Malvini. Aldemar, for his part, would watch from within the crowd, blending in with the villagers to avoid suspicion.

"Are you certain about this?" Aldemar had asked the night before, as they finalized details in the cabin that served as their temporary refuge.

Nicandro, still somewhat frail but with renewed fire in his eyes, nodded firmly.

"It's the only way. If we want the evidence to be credible, I must be the one to present it. My position within the Council will give it weight. You, Aldemar, must stay hidden. If they discover you, everything will be lost."

Though reluctant, Aldemar agreed. He knew his face was still being sought, and any misstep could ruin their cause.

On the day of the celebration, Aldemar mingled with the villagers, wrapped in a cloak that concealed his face. From a strategic vantage point, he kept his eyes on the main platform, where prominent nobles had gathered. As usual, Travius and Malvini occupied central positions, exuding a false generosity as they exchanged greetings and feigned concern for the welfare of the people.

Aldemar's heart raced as he saw Nicandro making his way through the crowd toward the platform. The elderly physician carried a small bag containing the evidence they had painstakingly gathered: altered sales records, incriminating correspondence, and bottles with residues of the poison used in the wells.

Despite his frailty, Nicandro climbed the platform steps with steady resolve, drawing curious glances from those present. Once before the crowd, his voice rang out, strong and defiant:

"Ladies and gentlemen, villagers of San Quirino! Today I must reveal a truth that has been hidden for far too long. The ones responsible for the illnesses that have plagued you and your families are here among us!"

A murmur swept through the plaza, filled with surprise and anticipation. Aldemar, watching from his position, kept his bow within reach. Though their plan was peaceful, he knew Nicandro's words would ignite a storm and wanted to be ready for anything.

The crowd, initially confused, fell silent. Travius, seated at the center, watched Nicandro with disdain.

"What nonsense are you spouting, old fool?" he asked with a sneering smile.

Nicandro held up the letters and bottles for all to see.

"Marquis Travius of the Hills and Duke Lorenzo Malvini have poisoned our wells to profit from the medicines they sell at unaffordable prices. Here is the proof! Their crimes are documented!" he declared, showing the sales records and explaining how the outbreaks coincided with the affected areas.

The murmur among the crowd kicked up again, louder than before. Travius, realizing the evidence was real, lost his composure.

"This is a farce!" he shouted, rising to his feet. "A fabrication from a bitter, resentful traitor! Nicandro, you've always been a coward, and now you dare to betray me?"

With a swift motion, he drew his sword and pointed it at Nicandro.

"You'll pay for this with your life!" he roared.

Unarmed and defenseless, Nicandro raised his hands in a calming gesture, but Travius, blinded by rage, lunged forward and struck a blow to his chest. The physician fell to his knees, wounded, as the crowd screamed in horror.

Aldemar, hidden in the throng, watched the scene unfold with his heart pounding. When he saw Travius raise his sword again, this time to deliver a fatal blow, he didn't hesitate. Drawing his bow, he swiftly nocked an arrow before letting it fly. The arrow cut through the air and struck Travius squarely in the chest, halting him mid-stride.

Staggering backward, The marquis' sword clattered to the platform as he fell. A deafening silence gripped the plaza. All eyes turned to the corrupt noble's lifeless body, the arrow still lodged in his chest. Beside him lay Nicandro, gravely wounded, clutching his bag of evidence as papers lay scattered on the platform.

Duke Lorenzo Malvini, frozen at first, quickly scanned the crowd and spotted Aldemar, still holding his bow. Pointing at him, he shouted:

"It was him! That traitor has killed Marquis Travius!"

The plaza erupted into chaos. The villagers, enraged by the truth that had been revealed, began to push against the few guards present. Malvini tried to escape, while Aldemar, knowing he had been exposed, slipped away into the crowd before the guards could apprehend him.

Amid the turmoil, a small group of brave villagers surrounded Nicandro, attempting to shield him from the guards who struggled to restore order. Unable to contain the mob, the soldiers eventually retreated along with Malvini and his entourage, leaving chaos in their wake.

The villagers carried Nicandro to a nearby cottage, along with the evidence they managed to collect and secure in his bag. There, they began treating him with the remedies Aldemar had taught them. His life hung by a thread, but his sacrifice had sparked the flames of rebellion.

Aldemar's Escape

"The path of the righteous is lonely, but never empty."
— Anonymous

Meanwhile, Baron Aldemar de Varenti ran toward the hills, his heart pounding. He knew his actions had made him a fugitive, but he felt no regret. He had protected Baron Nicandro and brought an end to Marquis Travius of the Hills, even if it meant losing everything.

In the shadows of the night, as the lights of the village faded behind him, Aldemar vowed that the fight was far from over. Though he was alone, the echo of his arrow reverberated like a promise: justice, though delayed, always finds its way.

The Spark of Rebellion

"The tree of resilience grows stronger in the storm."
— Anonymous

The death of Marquis Travius of the Hills had left a power vacuum and a mix of fear and indignation in San Quirino. While the nobles descended into panic at the growing unrest among the villagers, the peasants began to awaken from years of resignation. Stories of Travius' corruption and Duke Lorenzo Malvini's complicity spread like wildfire, fueled by long-simmering anger and discontent.

Nicandro remained gravely injured, hidden in the home of a peasant family that cared for him with unwavering devotion. Despite the guards' relentless efforts to track him down under Malvini's orders, the villagers—now fully aware of the Council's crimes—refused to cooperate.

Weak but lucid, Nicandro tried to stay informed of the developments through trusted villagers who visited him in secret.

"We must keep him hidden," insisted an elderly woman from the family sheltering him. "If they find him, they won't hesitate to kill him."

Nicandro nodded faintly, knowing that his survival depended on the loyalty and courage of the peasants who were risking everything to protect him.

Aldemar: A Fugitive on the Move

"Teaching is to touch a life forever."
— Henry Adams

Meanwhile, Baron Aldemar de Varenti continued his flight, moving from one village to another with the help of the same peasants he had once saved. He never stayed in one place for more than two days, knowing his capture would be inevitable if the guards under Duke Lorenzo Malvini's orders managed to track him. The villagers welcomed him with gratitude and respect, offering him shelter and food while ensuring he had a safe route to his next hiding place.

In every cottage where he found refuge, Aldemar used his time to teach families basic hygiene and prevention practices. His lessons were simple but effective: boil water before drinking it, keep wells clean, and avoid letting trash accumulate near homes. The villagers eagerly absorbed these teachings, grateful for the knowledge that gave them tools to protect themselves.

Despite the constant danger, Aldemar's resolve never wavered. He knew that Baron Nicandro's sacrifice and his own confrontation with Marquis Travius of the Hills had ignited a spark that could not be allowed to die out.

Part Three:
Rebellion Takes Shape

The People Organize

"The strength of a people lies not in their weapons, but in their will to change their destiny."
— Anonymous

The death of Marquis Travius of the Hills and the revelations of the Council's corruption had opened the eyes of the people. The peasants, who for generations had accepted their suffering as inevitable, began to organize. Small communities formed, dedicated to preventing disease and caring for one another. Wells were constantly monitored to prevent further contamination, and families shared the remedies Aldemar had taught them to prepare.

But the discontent went beyond health. The villagers were enraged by their living conditions: high tributes, lack of access to basic resources, and constant exploitation. The calls for justice grew louder by the day, soon becoming impossible to ignore. The rulers, unable to contain the growing rebellion, ordered the guards to intensify the search for Aldemar, hoping his capture would extinguish the flames of revolt.

The castle soldiers began searching every village and every home for the fugitive. They went door to door, interrogating families and inspecting potential hiding places. But the villagers, now united, remained loyal to Aldemar. Even when the guards' threats were clear, the answers were always the same:

"We don't know anything. We haven't seen anyone."

This improvised network of protection frustrated the soldiers and made it clear that the nobles' grip on the people was weakening. The peasants no longer feared as they once had, feeling empowered by the unity that Aldemar and Nicandro had inspired.

Moreover, their anger was no longer confined to whispers in the shadows. Meetings in the plazas became more frequent, and the villagers began demanding better living conditions and an end to oppression. Some, armed with farming tools, peacefully marched through the streets, shouting slogans that echoed against the castle walls. The nobles, accustomed to the people's submission, faced an unprecedented challenge.

Amid this chaos, Duke Lorenzo Malvini watched with growing concern. He knew his position was in jeopardy and that his only hope lay in capturing Aldemar to blame him for the unrest. But with each passing day, his control over the people continued to weaken.

From his hiding place, Aldemar heard rumors of the growing rebellion. Though he knew his capture was inevitable, he also understood that his sacrifice would not be in vain. He had planted the seed of change, and the peasants, united by a common cause, were willing to challenge the authorities for a fairer future.

"We don't need violence to show our strength; we will do this peacefully," Aldemar often said. "If we work together and care for our health, we will be stronger than any sword."

The improvements in the health and productivity of the communities became evident. Children laughed in the streets again, adults regained their strength, and the air of despair began to lift.

Meanwhile, Nicandro, still in hiding, was slowly recovering from his wounds. The families caring for him kept him informed about the progress of the rebellion, and though his body remained frail, his mind stayed sharp. He knew that the knowledge they had gathered and Aldemar's sacrifice were crucial to keeping the cause alive.

"Soon, I'll be ready to help again," he said one afternoon, struggling to rise from his bed. "I can't just sit here and do nothing."

An Unexpected Ally

"When the few unite for the common good,
they change the destiny of the many."
— Victor Hugo

News of Aldemar and Nicandro's activities began to spread not only among the peasants but also within noble circles. During an informal gathering, Lucian de Bellanti, Count of Bellanti, voiced his concerns about the rebellion he had heard of. Known for his inquisitive spirit and critical thinking, Lucian had always questioned the feudal model that thrived on the exploitation of peasants.

"I cannot understand how we can consider our position legitimate when it is built on the sickness and misery of those beneath us," Lucian declared during a dinner with his fellow young nobles.

Some regarded him with disdain, but others nodded silently. Among them, Princess Beatrice de Lorenzi, the daughter of a grand duke, voiced her support.

"If our fiefs had healthy, educated villagers, wouldn't they be more productive?" she remarked, glancing around the room. "A strong people make a strong fief."

Lucian saw an opportunity in her words and began gathering other nobles who shared his perspective. These younger nobles, less bound by the rigid traditions of their families, started discussing how social reforms could strengthen their lands rather than weaken them.

From these discussions the idea arose of secretly supporting Aldemar's cause. However, some hesitated, fearing the repercussions of defying the Council and figures like Duke Lorenzo Malvini.

The Betrayal of the Storm

"Courage is not in never falling, but in rising every time you fall."
— Confucius

On a dark and stormy night, as Aldemar rested in the home of a peasant woman in a remote village, a group of guards suddenly burst in, searching for the fugitive. The woman, brave and quick-witted, urgently woke Aldemar.

"Run! Go out the back. You don't have much time."

Grabbing his cloak and bow, Aldemar stepped into the cold, rain-soaked night. As he ran toward the hills, one of the guards spotted him.

"It's him! Catch him!" the guard shouted, pointing toward the silhouette vanishing into the downpour.

With his heart pounding, Aldemar sprinted up the nearby mountains, slipping over wet rocks and through branches that tore at his clothes. The storm raged around him, and the muddy ground grew treacherous.

As he tried to climb a steep incline, his foot slipped. Losing his grip, his body tumbled uncontrollably, crashing against rocks and roots until he lay motionless at the base of the hill.

The Capture

"Justice cannot be silenced with chains."
— Mahatma Gandhi

At dawn, the guards, weary but determined, found Aldemar unconscious and drenched. One of them checked his pulse and nodded.

"He's alive, but barely. Take him to the castle. This rebel will answer for his crimes."

Aldemar was chained and transported to the castle under heavy guard. The news of his capture spread rapidly, causing great unrest among the peasants and the nobles who secretly supported him.

Upon hearing of his capture, Lucian and Beatrice decided to act.

"We cannot let Aldemar face this alone. If they crush him, the rebellion will lose its strength," Lucian declared with resolve.

Beatrice nodded. "It's time for our words to become actions."

Meanwhile, in the villages, Aldemar's capture did not extinguish the spark of rebellion. The peasants, inspired by his sacrifice, continued to organize, guard their wells, and share knowledge. They knew their fight was just beginning, and though their leader was in the hands of his enemies, his legacy remained alive.

Part Four:
Justice and Resistance

The Voice of the People

"A wise ruler listens to the people; a foolish one silences them."
— Confucius

In the weeks following the capture of Baron Aldemar de Varenti, the rebellion grew into an unstoppable force. News of his teachings, the improved health of the villagers, and his courage in confronting Marquis Travius of the Hills reached the ears of His Serenity, the Doge of Venice, who initially responded with anger.

Protests and marches swelled, and the division among the nobles became increasingly apparent.

The Division Among the Nobles

"Nothing worth having is achieved without chaos."
— Friedrich Nietzsche

The family of Baron Nicandro, though divided, maintained secret contact with him. Among them, some supported the cause and saw Aldemar as a symbol of necessary change, while others viewed him as a threat to the established order.

"What Aldemar did was reckless and dangerous," a cousin of Nicandro remarked during a private meeting.

"And what do we have now?" retorted his sister, Baroness Flavia Renaldi, with conviction. "A rotten system that condemns the people to misery. Perhaps chaos is the price of change."

Nicandro, still weakened by his injuries, tried to mediate between the opposing views. He understood that the division among the nobles was a double-edged sword; it could weaken their enemies but also fragment the support they desperately needed.

Aldemar in the Cell

"A man may die, but his ideas live on forever."
— John F. Kennedy

Meanwhile, Aldemar remained in a dark, damp cell within the castle of Grand Duke Vittorio de Astelari, a noble known for his loyalty to the Republic of Venice and disdain for rebellions. Isolated and chained, Aldemar reflected on his fate. He knew his execution would not only serve as punishment but as a warning to the peasants, designed to sow fear among them.

The days were endless. The stone walls and the faint light that filtered through a small barred window constantly reminded him of his isolation. Yet, Aldemar felt no regret for his actions.

"If my death helps awaken the people, then it will not have been in vain," he murmured to himself.

Finally, the day of his trial arrived. In an improvised tribunal composed of nobles loyal to the Grand Duke and the Council, Aldemar was tried for the murder of Marquis Travius of the Hills. The charges were read aloud, and the verdict was delivered swiftly: death by hanging.

"Let this man serve as an example to those who dare to challenge the established order," declared the Grand Duke in a cold tone.

The People's Response

"Justice begins where fear ends."
— Mahatma Gandhi

Aldemar's death sentence only fueled the outrage of the peasants and the nobles who sympathized with his cause. Within days, a peaceful but substantial march was organized toward the palace of the Grand Duke in Astelari. Peasants from every village, carrying torches and makeshift banners, marched together, chanting:

"Justice for Aldemar! Down with the corrupt!"

The march, peaceful yet imposing, stretched for kilometers. Among the demonstrators, nobles like Count Lucian de Bellanti and Princess Beatrice de Lorenzi marched in disguise, showing their support without revealing their identities.

Upon reaching the Grand Duke's palace, the crowd gathered before the main gates, demanding the execution be annulled. The guards, vastly outnumbered, held their positions but showed visible signs of unease.

The Grand Duke's Dilemma

"The ruler who ignores the voice of their people will soon be silenced by it."
— Anonymous

From the high windows of the palace, Grand Duke Vittorio de Astelari watched the swelling crowd with growing concern. The protests had far exceeded his expectations, and the people's cries thundered through the air.

"My lord," one of his advisors murmured, leaning toward him, "we cannot ignore this demonstration. If we do, we risk a full-blown insurrection."

The Grand Duke slammed the table in frustration.

"We cannot allow the peasants to think they can dictate our decisions!" he roared. "But if we execute Aldemar, how long before these protests turn into an armed rebellion?"

The dilemma was clear: While yielding to the people's demands would show weakness, ignoring them could spark an even greater conflict.

The People's Trial

"The ruler who governs through fear will soon be governed by fear."
— Chinese Proverb

The square in front of Grand Duke Vittorio de Astelari's palace was a sea of torches and determined faces. Baron Nicandro, frail but resolute, leaned on a cane as he raised his voice above the crowd.

"Baron Aldemar de Varenti risked his life to save our children, to show us that we can live better!" he proclaimed, with a strength that seemed to surpass his weakened body. "We cannot let his sacrifice be in vain! We must demand justice and real change!"

The shouts of support and the agitation of the people swelled. Inside the palace, Grand Duke Vittorio de Astelari watched from a high window, surrounded by his advisors and local nobles. Among them stood Duke Lorenzo Malvini, his face pale and lips tightly pressed.

"This crowd is uncontrollable," Malvini said, struggling to maintain his composure. "We must bolster security before this turns into a full-scale revolt."

The Grand Duke slammed the table in frustration.

"We cannot hold them back with soldiers. If we act with force, this will become open war. Bring Aldemar here!" he commanded in a tone of authority. "Let him face the consequences of his actions before everyone."

The Arrival of Aldemar

"The strength of character is tested in adversity."
— Seneca

The guards dragged Baron Aldemar de Varenti, chained, from the depths of the castle to the square. His worn yet upright figure provoked a wave of shouts and cheers from the peasants. On the other side of the improvised platform, his father, Marquis Severino de Varenti, and his elder brother, Count Aldric de Varenti, watched with contrasting expressions: Severino with a mix of anger and disappointment, and Aldric with evident concern.

"This boy has brought shame upon us," Severino muttered to Aldric. "I cannot understand why you continue to support him."

Clenching his fists, Aldric replied in a low voice, "Because I see what you refuse to, Father. Aldemar is fighting for something greater than himself, something we, from within these walls, have ignored for far too long."

Aldemar ascended the platform under the watchful eyes of the crowd. Grand Duke Vittorio de Astelari, accompanied by Duke Lorenzo Malvini, addressed the people with a commanding tone.

"This man has defied the established order and killed a noble. His fate is sealed!"

Before the Grand Duke could continue, Nicandro, aided by two peasants, climbed onto the platform. Holding the evidence aloft, he raised his voice.

"Not so fast, Grand Duke Vittorio de Astelari! Before deciding Aldemar's fate, the people deserve to know the truth."

The crowd fell silent, waiting. Nicandro pointed directly at Malvini.

"This man, Duke Lorenzo Malvini, not only poisoned the wells of our villages to sicken our people and profit from overpriced medicines. He has also evaded taxes, robbing not only the people but also from the Republic of Venice!"

A wave of shock and fury swept through the square. Malvini tried to interject, but Nicandro gave him no opportunity.

"Here is the evidence!" he shouted, displaying transaction records and correspondence between Malvini and Travius. "This man has built his fortune on the misery of our people and the deception of His Serenity, the Doge of Venice!"

The Grand Duke, visibly uncomfortable, took the evidence and examined it. His expression hardened, but before he could act, Malvini stepped forward.

"This is a conspiracy!" he exclaimed, pointing at Nicandro and Aldemar. "This evidence is false—a desperate attempt by these traitors to cover their own crimes!"

The crowd erupted in anger, demanding justice. From among the masses came cries to investigate Malvini and release Aldemar. The situation was teetering on the edge of chaos.

Aldemar, who had remained silent until then, finally stood when the Grand Duke addressed him sternly.

"Aldemar, what do you have to say for yourself?"

"Grand Duke of Astelari," Aldemar began in a clear, unwavering voice, "how much longer will you ignore the voices of these people? If my life must end here, so be it. But if you kill me, you will not be killing a rebel, but a man who chose to fight for those you swore to protect."

His words momentarily quieted the tumult, but the Grand Duke remained undecided. Then Severino de Varenti stepped forward.

"This trial cannot proceed like this!" he exclaimed. "My son has brought shame to our family, but this is not justice. This is a spectacle."

Aldric, with a determination rarely seen, intervened.

"Father, perhaps it's time to listen to the people. They are not our enemies. If we continue to ignore their suffering, it will be our ruin."

The tension on the platform mounted. The cries of the peasants demanded justice not only for Aldemar but also for the exposure of Malvini's corruption. The Grand Duke glanced again at the evidence, then at the sea of angry but resolute faces.

Finally, he took a deep breath and, with a strong voice, announced:

"The execution is postponed until these accusations have been investigated!" he declared, turning to Malvini with a cold stare. "Duke Lorenzo Malvini, you are placed under arrest until the veracity of this evidence is confirmed."

The crowd erupted into cheers, though some murmured in uncertainty. While Aldemar was not freed, his execution had been stayed. The peasants knew their fight was far from over, but they had won a crucial battle that day.

As the guards escorted Malvini off the platform, the people continued chanting Aldemar's name. Though still in chains, he stood tall, knowing that his cause lived on in the hearts of those who supported him.

Part Five:
A New Order

The People's Protector

"The greatness of a ruler is measured by the prosperity of their people."
— Confucius

The news of Duke Lorenzo Malvini's arrest and the suspension of Baron Aldemar de Varenti's execution reached the Doge's Palace, where His Serenity, the Doge of Venice reside. What had begun as a whisper of rebellion among peasants had grown into a collective roar, echoing throughout the Most Serene Republic of Venice. Reports to the Doge detailed how villages that had adopted Aldemar's and Nicandro's teachings not only had healthier populations but were also becoming more productive. The local economy, driven by improved health and community cooperation, was beginning to thrive.

The King's Summons

"Great decisions are not easy, but their impact defines the course of history."
— Winston Churchill

Recognizing that the situation could no longer be ignored, His Serenety, the Doge of Venice, convened his Great Council. Among those present was Grand Duke Vittorio de Astelari, who, despite his initial opposition, presented the evidence against Malvini and highlighted the tangible benefits of Aldemar's actions.

"His Serenity," the Grand Duke said, bowing slightly, "though I have been strict in my previous stance, I must admit that this man's efforts have brought undeniable improvements to our lands. If we do not act wisely, we risk losing the trust of our people."

The Doge, initially angered by the villagers' defiance, now found himself confronted with undeniable results. As he listened to the reports of increased productivity and the improved quality of life among the villagers, his fury began to waver, giving way to a mix of curiosity and contemplation. These changes, though born of rebellion, hinted at something deeper—a potential path to greater prosperity for the Most Serene Republic of Venice. The Doge's expression softened slightly, but his tone remained firm.

"If Baron Aldemar's actions have been so impactful, why was he condemned?" the Doge asked, his gaze piercing the Great Council.

"For the death of Marquis Travius of the Hills, His Serenity," one of the advisors replied.

"Travius, in collusion with Duke Lorenzo Malvini, was deeply involved in corrupt activities. They poisoned village wells to create illness and then sold medicines at exorbitant prices while evading taxes imposed by the Most Serene Republic."

The Doge sat in silence for a moment, his expression unreadable. Finally, with a decisive gesture, he ordered:

"Bring Baron Aldemar to me. It is time to hear his story firsthand and make a decision that will ensure the stability of the Most Serene Republic."

The Royal Pardon

"The strength of a kingdom lies not in its walls,
but in the health and well-being of its people."
— Marcus Aurelius

Days later, Aldemar, still in chains, was brought before His Serenity. The Great Hall of the Doge's Palace was filled with nobles, many of whom had closely followed the rebellion. Among the crowd were Nicandro, recovering but present, and Marquis Severino de Varenti and Count Aldric de Varenti, watching on with mixed expressions.

The Doge fixed his gaze on the young noble.

"Baron Aldemar de Varenti, I have heard much about you. Some call you a traitor; others, a hero. What do you have to say in your defense?"

Standing tall despite his exhaustion, Aldemar spoke with unwavering conviction.

"His Serenety, I consider myself neither hero nor traitor. I simply did what I believe is right. The health of a people is the foundation of their strength. We cannot prosper while our people die from preventable diseases. If I am guilty of anything, it is fighting for them."

The Doge observed him silently, reflecting. Finally, he rose from his seat.

"Your cause is just, Baron Aldemar. Though your methods may have been questionable, the results are undeniable. By the power vested in me by the Most Serene Republic of Venice, you are granted pardon. But not only that."

The Great Hall of the Great Council fell into stunned silence. The Doge continued:

"I name you Protector of the Health of the Republic of Venice. You will be tasked with reforming our healthcare systems, ensuring that every man, woman, and child has access to clean water and medical treatment. It is a monumental challenge, but I trust you are prepared to face it."

The hall erupted in astonishment and applause. Aldemar, both surprised and humbled, bowed deeply.

"Thank you, His Serenety. I will not fail you."

News of this decision spread quickly with villages and towns celebrating spontaneously, seeing Aldemar's appointment as a symbol of hope and change.

"This is the beginning of something new!" said an elderly woman, hugging her grandson as she pointed toward the Doge's Palace. "At last, we have hope!"

Among the reformist nobles, Count Lucian Bellanti and Princess Beatrice Lorenzi exchanged knowing glances. They understood that the Most Serene Republic was at a crossroads, but Aldemar's appointment was a crucial step toward a more just future.

In the villages, the peasants continued organizing and applying Aldemar's teachings. Their unity grew, and the vision of a more equitable Most Serene Republic began to take shape. From the Doge's Palace, Aldemar, now serving as Protector of Health, knew that his true work was only just beginning.

A New Beginning

"The health of a nation is the reflection of its soul."
— Florence Nightingale

With his title as Protector of the Health of the Republic of Venice officialized by His Serenity, the Doge, Aldemar embarked on the ambitious task of building an inclusive and functional healthcare system. At his side, Baron Nicandro, now fully recovered, became his chief advisor, offering vast medical expertise and invaluable perspective. Nicandro was always grateful to Aldemar for saving his life.

Villages, organized into networks of mutual support, became the foundation of the new system. Prevention and health education were established as core principles. With the collaboration of reform-minded nobles such as Count Lucian Bellanti and Princess Beatrice Lorenzi, an unlikely yet effective coalition began to reshape the foundations of the Republic of Venice.

Resistance and Support

"True change is slow, but its fruits are sweet."
— African Proverb

Not all nobles embraced the reforms. Marquis Severino de Varenti, Aldemar's father, remained skeptical, fearing his son's actions could destabilize the delicate balance of the feudal system. Conversely, Count Aldric de Varenti, became his brother's strongest ally, showing a newfound perspective on the world.

"This will not be easy, brother," Aldric remarked one night as they reviewed a map of the kingdom, discussing plans to expand health programs. "Many are not ready for this change, but there's no doubt it is necessary."

Aldemar, with his usual calm demeanor, nodded.

"I know, Aldric," Aldemar replied calmly. "Yet each step we take, however small, improves someone's life. That is what matters. The desire for a dignified life is eternal, and we must guide it."

One afternoon, while overseeing the construction of a new aqueduct system in a nearby village, Aldemar and Nicandro shared a moment of reflection. Watching the peasants work side by side with engineers and apprentices, Nicandro quoted an old saying:

"Progress is like a river: strong and constant, but always facing stones in its path."

Aldemar smiled and calmly replied:

"And yet, the river never stops. It knows its destiny is to reach the sea."

The two men exchanged a look of understanding. Although they were fully aware of the challenges still ahead, they knew that change was real and the present was enough proof enough that the effort was worth it.

A Kingdom Transformed

"Nothing is permanent, except change."
— Heraclitus

Over time, the effects of the new healthcare system became evident throughout the Most Serene Republic. Disease rates dropped, productivity rose, and the sense of community among villagers strengthened. Even initially skeptical nobles began to recognize the benefits of the reforms.

Grand Duke Vittorio de Astelari, who had closely monitored Aldemar's progress, acknowledged the young baron's impact during a meeting in the Great Council.

"Though I doubted this young baron at first, I must admit his vision and determination have brought prosperity where there was once despair."

The recognition of figures like the Grand Duke, combined with growing popular support, cemented Aldemar's position as a transformative leader.

In his residence, Marquis Severino de Varenti watched in silence. Though he did not openly express it, he began to see in his son something he had always desired but never fully understood: the ability to lead with true purpose.

The Serenity Republic of Venice was changing. While the path to a more just future was long, the current of progress flowed strongly, guided by Baron Aldemar de Varenti, Nicandro, and their allies. His Serenity, the Doge, in his pragmatism, had bet on innovation, and the people strengthened became the greatest guarantee of a prosperous and united realm. For how long? No one knew. What they did know was that they were far better off than before.

"Everything flows; nothing remains."
— Heraclitus

Reality is in constant flux. While the permanence of any situation is uncertain, the transformations that lead to a better state are worth recognizing and nurturing.

www.ingramcontent.com/pod-product-compliance
Lightning Source LLC
Chambersburg PA
CBHW070649130626
46555CB00006B/2782